NEXT TIME THERE'S A PANDEMIC

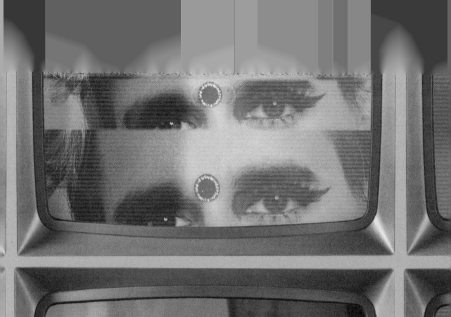

NEXT TIME THERE'S A PANDEMIC

CLC Kreisel Lecture Series

VIVEK SHRAYA

Published by

University of Alberta Press
1–16 Rutherford Library South
11204 89 Avenue NW
Edmonton, Alberta, Canada T6G 2J4
Amiskwacîwâskahican | Treaty 6 |
Métis Territory
uap.ualberta.ca

and

Canadian Literature Centre /
Centre de littérature canadienne
3–5 Humanities Centre
University of Alberta
Edmonton, Alberta, Canada T6G 2E5
www.abclc.ca

LIBRARY AND ARCHIVES CANADA
CATALOGUING IN PUBLICATION

Title: Next time there's a pandemic / Vivek
    Shraya.
Names: Shraya, Vivek, 1981– author. |
Canadian Literature Centre, issuing body.
Series: Henry Kreisel lecture series.
Description: Series statement: CLC Kreisel
    lecture series
Identifiers: Canadiana (print) 20210347554 |
    Canadiana (ebook) 20210347570 |
    ISBN 9781772126051 (softcover) |
    ISBN 9781772126082 (EPUB) |
    ISBN 9781772126099 (PDF)
Subjects: LCSH: Shraya, Vivek, 1981– |
    LCSH: COVID-19 Pandemic, 2020– —
    Anecdotes. | LCGFT: Creative nonfiction.
Classification: LCC PS8637.H73 N49 2022 |
    DDC C818/.603—dc23

First edition, first printing, 2022.
First printed and bound in Canada by
Houghton Boston Printers, Saskatoon,
Saskatchewan.
Copyediting and proofreading by
Joanne Muzak.

University of Alberta Press is committed to
protecting our natural environment. As part
of our efforts, this book is printed on Enviro
Paper: it contains 100% post-consumer
recycled fibres and is acid- and chlorine-free.

The Canadian Literature Centre acknowledges
the support of Dr. Eric Schloss and the
Faculty of Arts for the CLC Kreisel Lecture
delivered by Vivek Shraya in March 2021
online through the University of Alberta.

University of Alberta Press gratefully
acknowledges the support received for its
publishing program from the Government
of Canada, the Canada Council for the Arts,
and the Government of Alberta through the
Alberta Media Fund.

To the lives lost to the HIV/AIDS pandemic.

FOREWORD
The CLC Kreisel Lecture Series

THE CANADIAN LITERATURE CENTRE (CLC) was established in 2006, thanks to the leadership gift of noted Edmontonian bibliophile Dr. Eric Schloss. The Kreisel Lecture Series is an annual event dedicated to nurturing public as well as scholarly engagement with the pressing concerns of writers in Canada. This series was established in honour of Professor Henry Kreisel. Author, University Professor, and Officer of the Order of Canada, Kreisel was born into a Jewish family in Vienna in 1922. He left his homeland for England in 1938 and was interned in Canada for eighteen months during the Second World War. After studying at the University of Toronto, he was hired in 1947 to teach at the University of Alberta, where he served as Chair of English from 1961 to 1970. He served as Vice-President (Academic) from 1970 to 1975, when he was named University Professor, the highest scholarly award bestowed on its faculty members by the University of Alberta. An inspiring and beloved teacher who taught generations of students to love literature, Professor Kreisel was among the first to champion Canadian literature in university classrooms and to bring the experience of immigrants to modern Canadian literature. His works include two novels, *The Rich Man* (1948) and *The Betrayal* (1964), and a collection of short stories, *The Almost Meeting* (1981). His internment diary, alongside critical essays on his writing, appears in *Another Country: Writings by and about Henry Kreisel* (1985). He died in Edmonton in 1991. The generosity and foresight of Professor Kreisel's teaching at the University of Alberta continues to inspire the CLC in its research pursuits, public outreach, and continued commitment to the ever-growing richness, complexity, and diversity of literatures in Canada.

The Kreisel Lectures showcase how writers help us understand the textures of life in this country. Each year, an established author is invited to speak about an issue that is important to them, whether because it is close to their heart, foundational to their experience, or pressing and of-the-moment; often, it is all of these things at once. The series includes lectures about Indigenous resurgence, oppression and social justice, cultural identity, place and displacement, the spoils of history, storytelling, censorship, language, reading in a digital age, literary history, personal memory, and, now, the necessity of art during a pandemic. Usually delivered to a live audience on the University of Alberta campus, located on Treaty 6 Territory and Region 4 of the Métis Nation of Alberta, the Kreisel Lectures frequently also air to audiences across Canada as episodes on CBC Radio's *Ideas*. All of the lectures become books like this one, published in partnership with University of Alberta Press.

During the COVID-19 pandemic, nothing at the CLC could happen in the usual way. We were tremendously lucky to have the innovative and talented Vivek Shraya as the 2021 Kreisel Lecturer. Shraya is a prolific multimedia artist and writer as well as an important community leader and mentor. The founder of the publishing imprint VS. Books, through which she offers mentorship and publishing opportunities to Indigenous and Black writers and writers of colour in Canada, she is also a director on the board of the Tegan and Sara Foundation, whose mission is to improve the lives of LGBTQ+ women and girls. Her award-winning work ranges across literature, film, and music, frequently combining all three in arresting ways.

Artists like Shraya remind us of the importance of play. Artists and writers are creators: experimenting at the boundaries of genre, testing the limits of form, defying and exceeding our expectations, they give expression to a very human need for playfulness that expands the worlds we inhabit. Breaking up the habitual was precisely what many of us needed after more than a year of living under pandemic restrictions. When it became clear that, for the first time ever, the Kreisel Lecture would have to take place online, Shraya harnessed all of her creative and collaborative energy to produce something truly unique and special. This book expands on the innovative filmed lecture (which can still be viewed on the CLC's website), which reflects on the constraints of living in the pandemic and what she would do differently "next time." *Next Time There's a Pandemic* demonstrates why, as Shraya insists, "art is essential."

Shraya's online Kreisel Lecture was presented in March 2021 with an interactive introduction with J. R. Carpenter, an award-winning artist, writer, and researcher working across performance, print, and digital media, and the University of Alberta's 2020– 2021 Writer in Residence. Their conversation has also been expanded here as an Afterword.

SARAH WYLIE KROTZ
Interim Director, Canadian Literature Centre
Edmonton, June 2021

LIMINAIRE

La collection des conférences Kreisel CLC

LE CENTRE DE LITTÉRATURE CANADIENNE a été créé en 2006 grâce au don directeur du bibliophile illustre edmontonien, le docteur Eric Schloss. La série de Conférences Kreisel est un événement annuel consacré à l'engagement du public et des universitaires face aux préoccupations urgentes des auteurs et autrices au Canada. Cette série de conférences a été créée en l'honneur du professeur Henry Kreisel. Auteur, professeur d'université et officier de l'Ordre du Canada, Kreisel est né à Vienne d'une famille juive en 1922. Il a quitté son pays natal pour l'Angleterre en 1938 et a été interné au Canada pendant dix-huit mois lors de la Seconde Guerre mondiale. Après ses études à l'Université de Toronto, il devient professeur à l'Université de l'Alberta en 1947, et à partir de 1961 jusqu'à 1970 il a dirigé le Département d'anglais. De 1970 à 1975, il a été vice-recteur (universitaire), et a été nommé professeur hors rang en 1975, la plus haute distinction scientifique décernée par l'Université de l'Alberta à un membre de son professorat. Professeur adoré, il a transmis l'amour de la littérature à plusieurs générations d'étudiants, et il a été parmi les premiers écrivains modernes du Canada à aborder l'expérience immigrante. Son œuvre comprend les romans, *The Rich Man* (1948) et *The Betrayal* (1964), et un recueil de nouvelles intitulé *The Almost Meeting* (1981). Son journal d'internement, accompagné d'articles critiques sur ses écrits, paraît dans *Another Country: Writings by and about Henry Kreisel* (1985). Il est décédé à Edmonton en 1991. La générosité et la prévoyance de l'enseignement du professeur Kreisel à l'Université de l'Alberta continuent d'inspirer le CLC dans ses activités de recherche, sa sensibilisation du public et son engagement envers la richesse, la complexité et la diversité toujours croissantes des écrits au Canada.

Les conférences Kreisel font preuve du fait que la création littéraire nous aide à comprendre le tissu de la vie dans ce pays. Chaque année, un.e invité.e s'exprime sur un sujet qui lui tient à cœur, que ce soit parce qu'il est à la base de son expérience ou qu'il est urgent et actuel; souvent il s'agit des deux à la fois. La série se compose de conférences sur la résurgence autochtone, l'oppression et la justice sociale, l'identité culturelle, le lieu et le déplacement, les dépouilles de l'histoire, la narration, la censure, la langue, la lecture à l'ère numérique, l'histoire littéraire, la mémoire personnelle et maintenant: la nécessité de l'art pendant une pandémie. Habituellement présentées à un auditoire en direct sur le campus de l'Université de l'Alberta, situé sur le territoire du Traité 6 et de la Région 4 de la Nation Métis, les Conférences Kreisel sont fréquemment diffusées à des auditoires partout au Canada sous forme d'épisodes diffusées par "IDEAS" de la radio CBC. Les conférences sont aussi publiées sous forme des livres comme celui que vous tenez en main, en collaboration avec University of Alberta Press.

Pendant la pandémie de COVID-19, rien au CLC ne pouvait se passer de manière habituelle. Nous avons eu énormément de chance d'avoir l'innovatrice et la talentueuse Vivek Shraya comme conférencière Kreisel 2021. Shraya est une artiste et écrivaine multimédia prolifique ainsi qu'une importante dirigeante et mentore communautaire. La fondatrice de la maison d'édition VS. Books, à travers laquelle elle offre du mentorat et des opportunités de publication aux artistes littéraires autochtones et racisé.e.sr au Canada, Shraya est également directrice au conseil d'administration de la Fondation Tegan and Sara, dont la mission est d'améliorer la vie des femmes et des filles LGBTQ+.

Son travail primé recouvre la littérature, le cinéma et la musique, combinant fréquemment les trois de manière saisissante.

Les artistes comme Shraya nous rappellent l'importance du jeu. Les artistes créent: expérimentant aux frontières des genres, testant les limites de la forme, défiant et dépassant nos attentes, ces artistes expriment le besoin très humain du jeu qui élargit les mondes que nous habitons. Rompre avec l'habitude était précisément ce dont beaucoup d'entre nous avions besoin après plus d'un an de pandémie. Lorsqu'il est devenu clair que, pour la première fois, la conférence Kreisel devait avoir lieu en ligne, Shraya a mobilisé toute son énergie créative et collaborative pour produire quelque chose de vraiment unique et spécial. Ce livre développe la conférence filmée novatrice (qui peut toujours être visionnée sur le site Web du CLC), et réfléchit aux contraintes de la vie pendant la COVID et à ce que nous pourrions faire différemment une prochaine fois. *Next Time There's a Pandemic* démontre pourquoi, comme le souligne Shraya, «l'art est essentiel».

La Conférence Kreisel de Vivek Shraya a été présentée en mars 2021 avec une introduction ludique et interactive par J. R. Carpenter, une artiste, écrivaine et chercheuse primée travaillant dans les domaines de la performance, des presses écrites et numériques et comme écrivaine-en-résidence 2020−21 à l'Université de l'Alberta. Leur conversation a donné lieu à la postface de ce livre.

SARAH WYLIE KROTZ
Directrice par intérim, Centre de littérature canadienne
Edmonton, juin 2021

NEXT TIME THERE'S A PANDEMIC

AFTER THE LOCKDOWN ENDED IN JUNE 2020, I was grateful
when massage clinics re-opened. While I prefer a silent massage,
the pandemic had already tested the limits of my introversion,
so I willingly engaged in the requisite chit chat about lockdown
experiences with my therapist during my first post-lockdown
massage. He gushed behind his mask: "Oh man. It was so great.
Every day I woke up, drank coffee, read, rode my bike..."

I had no idea how to respond (and was thankful that my
head was hanging in the face cradle). My therapist's description
did sound pretty great. But it was nothing like my own anxiety-
ridden ordeal of struggling to do my job (which requires me to
be creative), binge watching TV, and worrying incessantly about
loved ones, the world, and the future.

Had I done the lockdown wrong?

| It's December 2020. Alberta is reaching record highs for
COVID-19 cases. The highly anticipated second wave is here in
full force. But so far, there is no second lockdown. Mall, casino,
and restaurant doors are all wide open. Not even a deadly virus
will keep this province away from raking in big Christmas bucks.

Though I tend to be existential all year long, December
is typically a time of reflection, evaluation, and anticipation

for me. I review the previous year's resolutions and my list of accomplishments with gratitude, and then mentally draft a new list of goals for the coming year. I ask myself how I can be and do better.

When I review my December 2019 lists, it appears as though I was standing on the edge of what was looking like one of the busiest and most exciting years of my artistic career. In January 2020, I was going to launch my first play, *How to Fail as a Popstar*, as a workshop in Calgary, and then fly to Toronto to perform a two-week run of the show in February 2020. My theatre debut would be swiftly followed by the April 2020 launch of my second novel, *The Subtweet*, a project I was especially looking forward to releasing because of the many barriers I had faced in bringing it to life. I had booked a cross-country tour, and even created a custom tour uniform for the occasion (as I always do). In May 2020, my play was scheduled to have its international debut in Germany—one of my first opportunities in my two-decade-long art career to perform in Europe—with the hope of soliciting further bookings from other international programmers. In September 2020, I was set to launch the ten-year anniversary edition of my first book, *God Loves Hair*, which I originally self-published. The celebration of this milestone would be accompanied by my second cross-Canadian tour of the year. In October 2020, I would return to Germany, this time as an honoured delegate at the prestigious Frankfurt Book Fair, another rare opportunity to introduce myself and my work (this time, my writing) to the European market, and hopefully garner interest in future translations of my books. And in between all of these releases and events, opportunities I hadn't planned or predicted would no doubt have emerged.

2020 played out wildly different than any of us could have imagined. I did get to perform my play in Calgary and Toronto— the timing of which now seems miraculous, given that had it been scheduled even a week or so later the turnout could have been drastically reduced and shows, or even the entire run, could have been cancelled. Given that theatre re-opening dates continue to get pushed back, and programming continues to get shuffled, it's hard to say when, if ever, I'd get another opportunity to debut my play, let alone perform it again. I did release the two books but obviously all of the scheduled live events were cancelled. For books published by small presses especially, as mine were, general public awareness and sales of new releases are inextricably tied to the personal connections made with audiences on tour, so the toll of these lost opportunities is incalculable. And, after years of wishing I could spend less time on the road and more time at home, where I could be still and focus on creating, I found out the hard way that stillness and isolation isn't all that inspiring for me. That a huge part of my creative force comes from connecting with other humans, hearing their responses to my work, and engaging with other artists and their work—all vital experiences for my job that I wasn't able to have.

Artists traffic in a mystical, intangible element called "momentum"—the energy of interest that follows a new project, if the stars align (also known as "buzz" or "hype"). The general equation is: momentum = future opportunities (and conversely, lack of momentum = shortage of future opportunities). You can't put a price on momentum, nor can it be postponed or recreated. Instead, any of the momentum I had accumulated in my pre-pandemic art career, leading up to and during my play run, disappeared when the March 2020 lockdown began. I will never know where else I might have performed my play, how different the response to my books might have been, the new audiences I could have reached, what impact my art could have had, the growth and turns my career could have made if the pandemic had not occurred.

Boohoo, right? In the face of staggering global rates of illness and death, thinking, let alone talking (or writing) about career or personal losses feels shameful. I spent most of 2020 silently trying to suffocate the disappointment and grief I felt about the aforementioned losses while simultaneously berating myself for being so fucking selfish.

Unfortunately, it doesn't seem like there's much to look forward to in the year ahead. Despite the reports that vaccines are coming, 2021 looks like it's going to be a bad sequel to 2020. More of the same. More holding pattern.

For me, this means another year of seeing my families—chosen and biological—rarely, if at all, a calendar of scattered bookings for live event that realistically will not happen, and hours spent crawling further down IMDB, Rotten Tomatoes, and Taste Dive for TV and movie ideas that I have not yet pursued (this month: action flicks starring a hairy Baldwin brother). Another year of feeling like less of a working artist and even less of a human—at best, a waste of resources, and at worst, a carrier for a virus.

Unable to look forward clearly or optimistically, I find myself looking backward critically, wondering what I would do differently if I had to live through 2020 all over again, the pandemic over again. And reflecting on what I wish we had collectively done differently.

Here are five of my reflections.

1
STAY
CARING

AS THE NOVEL CORONAVIRUS SPREAD in early 2020, COVID-specific words and phrases like "PPE," "social distancing," and "flatten the curve" became ubiquitous. I personally hope I never hear the word "unprecedented" again. Another early phrase I found vexing was "stay safe."

As a writer and English teacher, obsessing over and being critical about word choice is my job (don't get me started on the biggest coronavirus plot twist: not so "novel" after all!), and yet I was initially unable to figure out why "stay safe" bothered me. It may seem finicky to harp on a well-intentioned phrase, but as our social interactions were reduced so drastically, this phrase was often the only message I would hear from anyone other than my boyfriend. The more I was urged to "stay safe," the more aware I became that that safety isn't something that everyone has access to or can choose. This awareness was acute especially because, ironically, I heard this phrase most frequently from grocery clerks and delivery people, some of the many workers who were forced to risk their health to survive and so that *others* could survive. Were they actually encouraging me to stay safe, or was this phrase a kind of mantra for themselves? Or were they (subconsciously) pleading with me to stay *home* to avoid endangering them?

The general interchangeable usage of "stay safe" and "stay home" also implied that home is a safe place, a haven for everyone. But the increase of domestic violence during COVID is a reminder that this assumption isn't true. For people faced with this reality, "stay safe" is an ignorant and even callous directive.

Personally, I can try to stay as safe as I want, but as a trans feminine, queer, brown person, regardless of whether there is a global crisis, I can't control how others react to me. Pre-pandemic, I approached any kind of outdoor activity, including walking, with a baseline of trepidation and alertness because of my past experiences of public harassment. I'm already used to walking on the edge of the sidewalk, or the grass, or even the road when other people are around, not because I was previously scared of catching a virus, but so that men behind me can pass, or rather so I'm never walking with a man directly behind me.

Perhaps related: I spotted a number of openly affectionate queer couples on my daily pandemic walks, an uncommon sight, and I wondered if queers felt safer to express themselves publicly with so many (straight) people forced to be indoors.

Next time there's a pandemic, I hope that whatever "slogan" we use is less about individual responsibility, like "stay safe" or even "take care," and more about collective care and action, like "stay caring" or "stay kind." More importantly, I hope we will consider how we can *provide* collective care, especially when physical contact with others is restricted.

For me, this meant thinking beyond the sanctioned contact of biological family and romantic partners. I made a conscious effort to centre those in my life who had the least support—my single women friends—by phoning them regularly or sending them gift cards for essential goods and services. Similarly, friends sent me care packages and flowers, and some also dropped off baked goods. Some of us had transparent conversations about the challenge of wanting to check in regularly while understanding how impossible it felt at times to come up with an adequate response to "How are you?" One solution was to send each other daily heart emojis to communicate caring and as "proof of life."

I also tried to remember those outside my social circles and by supporting local businesses, donating to community organizations, like women's shelters, and contacting members of Parliament to lobby for wage increases for frontline workers.

But as I navigated my own mental health, most of my efforts were sporadic at best, and seldom felt adequate.

2
SKIP THE GRATITUDE AND SAY WHAT YOU FEEL

THROUGHOUT 2020, I also heard many versions of the comment that only those who are willing to adapt will endure. These comments were directed not just toward business owners and arts administrators but also at individuals. The subtext: *survival of the fittest*.

The problem with survival of the fittest is that it glorifies individual strength while refusing to acknowledge the factors that enable some individuals to be "stronger" than others. Quarantining with my white, straight-passing boyfriend, I was constantly reminded of my lack of emotional strength. He commented early in the pandemic that he could likely quarantine for months and months and be fine. Even be content. And he truly did seem unphased by the chaos, peacefully watching movies and playing video games while I paced around our place or forced myself to write or read (but my eyes refusing to lock into any of the words).

Witnessing his apparent "adaptation," I wondered what was wrong with me. What was my problem? Why couldn't I figure the pandemic out (because it was a puzzle, right?)? Why couldn't I settle into a stable and productive routine even after months had passed? I had a stable income, a beautiful apartment, supportive friends. I was not in immediate danger but I still felt on edge.

It took me awhile to realize that this unease stemmed from the reality that, despite the repeated insistence that "we're all in this together," we all didn't enter the pandemic equally. The panic of the lockdown exacerbated the physical and mental effects of my previous experiences of trauma and oppression. Every night I dreamt of being hunted or killed, or I had unimaginative stress dreams about arriving late (and pantless) on the first day of class. When I was awake, my inability to exert control over my life, which is one of my primary survival mechanisms, left me in freefall, endlessly worrying about the end of my art career, as dozens of my gigs were instantly cancelled, and about being fired from my teaching job, as the institution where I work (and am the newest department hire) continued to announce drastic budget cuts. I also worried because my chronic pain is triggered by computer work, so I was unable to transition to online teaching without causing further physical harm and I didn't know what impact this would have on my job security. Or rather, what would it take for me to feel secure, when being trans (and racialized) is associated with unemployment? Any security I have acquired has always been anomalous, not the norm, for someone like me. In contrast, my white colleagues (thankfully) reassured me multiple times that our jobs were safe. I wondered what it would be like to possess that kind of certainty and conviction in the midst of precarity. Is it surprising, then, that a white man can quarantine and be content compared to those of us whose identities are more stringently tied to familial and social responsibilities or whose experiences have taught us the necessity of living in a state of constant anticipation of danger?

As someone who struggles to manage the effects oppression has on my mental health, I have a finely tuned system that keeps me afloat. I routinely work out to expend my excess anxiety. I go out to see movies in a theatre at least once a week to get out of my brain and away from my phone (and task list) for two hours. I see my therapist once every few months. And as I mentioned earlier, I regularly go for massages. For me, massages are not only a means of relaxing, but also a way to temporarily alleviate my chronic pain.

When lockdowns have been debated by our government, the objections typically focus on the economic impact: the harm done to businesses or business owners. But for me, the lockdown meant that suddenly I couldn't access any of my mental health supports. Gyms, theatres, and health practitioners' offices all closed abruptly and indefinitely (I did try Zooming with my therapist, but our conversations hit a wall of "it's not you, it's the pandemic," which was validating at first, but then about as useful and motivating as a quote I read in a CBC article about chronic stress in the pandemic: "The way to solve boredom during the pandemic is to end the pandemic." Easy. In fairness to my therapist, I assume her training did not prepare her to provide strategies for dealing with a pandemic.) So of course, my coping mechanisms deteriorated, which deepened my melancholy and sense of purposelessness. My thoughts of suicide ballooned from a few times a year to a few times a month.

The lockdown also made it impossible to spend time with loved ones, but I made an effort to reach out frequently.

Hey, how's it going?

Fine, I guess? My parents are safe. The family is ok. Our health is ok. You know, working from home is an adjustment but I am grateful to have a job...I can't complain.

Does this sound familiar? This is how most of my conversations in 2020 started. Everyone parroted their gratitude/privilege list as a response to "How are you?" Expressing gratitude is a useful practice in re-establishing perspective and listing privileges can also be an important endeavour if it leads to thinking about how you might deploy them to support others who have less. But what concerned me is that no would actually tell me *how they were doing*. Consequently, I didn't have a real sense of how my loved ones were coping, which also meant I wasn't able to support them as much or as specifically as I wanted.

I tried to encourage friends to skip this intro, inviting them to discuss their feelings with me honestly and directly. No one took the option. Living with the looming threat of illness and death, no one wanted to complain about their less-than-dire circumstances because "it could be worse." And no one wanted to be a burden during a time when everyone already seemed overburdened.

What this silence meant for me, as someone who couldn't access any of my usual mental health supports and who also used the gratitude/privilege list as a form of deflection, is that a pile of unexpressed emotions started to build. Because when you feel "bad" and you don't acknowledge the feeling somehow, there's no chance for the bad feeling to be seen and to dissipate. So the feeling grows.

Because I was unable to communicate my thoughts and feelings fully—not assume that others wouldn't judge me for expressing how I really felt—I began to avoid my friends, to stop responding to their texts and calls, and at times to resent them. My emotional isolation increased my paranoia that everyone else was coping with the pandemic better than I was. Another way that the survival of the fittest mentality impacted me was that I didn't want to appear weak and was afraid of being left behind. I'm embarrassed to admit that I even enviously accused a friend of "thriving" after observing her spurt of productivity.

But there were a handful of moments when I finally let go, let my words and feelings flood out while talking to a friend. Despite these disclosures being less conscious choices to share my thoughts and more acts of desperation and disintegration, and also didn't exactly result in "feeling better" after, I did feel a release, incrementally lighter. These moments also allowed my friends to remind me that I was loved, which, sadly, was easy to forget this year. And while love isn't always a cure or salve, it made the hours after a little more bearable.

Next time there's a pandemic, let's try not to wait to have a breakdown before we talk about our emotions with our friends. Let's reach out actively, skip the gratitude/privilege list and say what we feel to each other. Let's trust that the people who love us *want* to hear us, and can manage their own struggles while listening to ours—and will let us know when they can't. Or let's ask each other directly, as my friends and I learned to do this year, with questions like, "Do you have the capacity for a phone call today?" or "Do you have time and energy to talk now?" Because in the absence of mental health resources, talking openly to one another might be the only support we have, and is crucial in preserving and potentially strengthening our relationships, especially with the loss of physical proximity.

3
NOTHING IS BETTER THAN SOMETHING

SOMETIMES WHEN I'M ON MY PHONE shooting off work emails and texts while I am out for a walk or when I'm in the bathroom or car, the biggest capitalist con of the 2000s seems to be the way that we were tricked into buying expensive little computers to carry around with us so that we can work all the time—all under the guise of being more connected to each other. The pandemic capitalized on this foundation of constant "connection" and took it to a whole new level as suddenly we were not just working from home, but rather the home became the office.

As someone who regularly worked from home before the pandemic, this, in theory, shouldn't have felt like a significant change. But when my partner also began working from home and needed a quiet place to make confidential phone calls, I had to give up my home office. The kitchen, living room area, and even the bedroom became my part-time workspaces, which meant there was nowhere in our apartment that didn't remind me of work, or that offered a respite from work. Of course, we were privileged to have the option to work from home. But when large sectors of people are working from home, not only do the lines between work and home become blurry, but our experiences of *time* also got blurred. How often did I hear someone ask rhetorically, "What is a weekend?" I now frequently get work emails on the weekend.

When the lockdown started, the first impact it had on my job was that the spring book tour for my novel *The Subtweet* was cancelled. This was actually a joint book tour, with two other authors launching new books with a different publisher than mine, with nine stops hosted by various festivals and bookstores. Given the many parties involved, this tour took half a year to assemble. Before I even had time to process its cancellation, virtual events sprouted around me. Initially I asserted, "There's no way in hell that you'll see me doing that Zoom shit." While I can appreciate a DIY aesthetic (and also recognize that sometimes DIY is not so much a choice, but more about economic limitations), I've always placed high value on producing polished work. And by polished, I'm not just referencing my perfectionist tendencies, nor do I mean "expensive-looking," but an overall thoughtfulness around presentation that seemed to vanish in the virtual space. It still pains me that a year in, technical difficulties during virtual events are accepted as the norm, and that a glitch-free virtual event is anomalous. Thankfully, my publishers assured me that there would likely be live opportunities to promote my book in the fall.

But after following the chaotic news stream and the endless speculation in my feed for a few days, I worried if there would even be a fall without the coronavirus. We seemed to know so little about it. So I dove in, spent hours researching lighting and audio, and re-launched the book tour—a virtual edition, cobbled together in just a week with the spirited help of my publicist and several bookstores and festivals. Throughout this process, I told myself, "It's better to do something instead of nothing" and treated this preparation process and the events themselves as a new experiment in my career. "Live events? Been there, done that," was my temporary positive-thinking reframe.

And I'm glad I changed my mind. It felt somewhat fitting to promote a book about the internet via the internet. I was fortunate that so many people tuned in for the six events (partly because this was early enough in the pandemic that "Zoom fatigue" hadn't yet kicked in, or even been named). While their virtual presence didn't replace the energy of live events, it was interesting to experience a different form of real-time feedback, as a peer pointed out, to see what attendees were thinking *while* they were thinking it, through their comments and emojis in the chat. I also was momentarily captivated by the process of learning which online platforms were more conducive for attendance and engagement and provided the most options and freedom for the presenter, and passionately compiled these stats for myself and my publisher. And ultimately, my suspicions were right: in-person book events, like most cultural gatherings, didn't return in the fall.

"It's better to do something instead of nothing" has been my guiding principle since this tour, carrying me through the rest of 2020. But now, at the end of the year, as I look ahead to 2021, I'm exhausted by the ongoing process of rebooking of gigs followed by relentless cancellations and by the accompanying pressure to pivot—another word I have grown to loathe—by re-imagining and recreating many of these live events or other forms of art for a virtual context. While many artists have been able to find creative ways to pivot, to share art online, I'm not entirely sure whether recording my work and throwing it on the internet is creating art or creating content. As the pandemic restrictions dragged on, it seemed like both artists and businesses became increasingly obsessed with creating content, because "everyone is at home sitting on their phones."

In fairness to artists, I know too well and sympathize with the pressure to be constantly visible, and constantly visibly producing in this digital-24/7-all-access era, to maintain and increase one's following and to avoid slipping into obscurity. But I feel a little less clear about the intentions of institutions during this time. For instance, when festivals approached me about live-streaming my play on their platforms, I had difficulty discerning whether I was reluctant because this wasn't what was best for the art—that I had deliberately created for a live audience—or if I was being unnecessarily inflexible and unimaginative about the new possibilities of online dissemination, or if the invitations were, in part, a way for organizations to maintain and project a sense of relevance, to give audiences and funders something rather than nothing. Did they genuinely respect my work and want to support me or was my art merely content for them? What might have happened if more organizations had opted not to push for (sometimes overly ambitious) virtual programming, especially given waning audience interest, and the burnout the workers at these organizations were experiencing as they worked to pivot while simultaneously managing massive institutional cuts and changes?

While many people did not have the option to choose to do nothing (or even to do less) during the lockdown, for those who do, it seems worth questioning if there are times when it's better— or at least just as worthy and perhaps even humane—to do nothing rather than something?

I wish I had approached every request to virtually pivot by first asking myself:

Do you actually want to do this?
Do you have the emotional capacity to do this?
Will you be creating something meaningful and beautiful?

These questions helped guide me in embracing the opportunity to make something creative for this year's Kreisel Lecture—an animated, multimedia video, instead of yet another Zoom event.

In 2021 I'm telling myself that it's ok if I don't post as often, if I generate less content, or even make less art if I don't feel inspired. That the line between art and compromise is sometimes not worth crossing, even for the sake of so-called adaptation.

4
VALUE ARTISTS

THE CLASSIFICATION OF SPECIFIC TYPES OF WORK, and by extension specific groups of workers, as "essential" during the pandemic highlighted what I have always suspected: as an artist, my work is not essential. I'm not being self-deprecating. I know that I am fortunate to be a working artist. I spent a lot of 2020 grappling with whether it is possible to still be of service somehow, to contribute meaningfully to my communities, when the work I do isn't essential.

As I was contemplating my own value as a worker, I noticed that the value of my work within the systems around me was being depreciated, perhaps because some saw an opportunity to capitalize on the desperation of artists who had lost gig income. I started getting offered gigs that paid fifty dollars, a fraction of what I had been paid for gigs just months prior. When I calculate the three hours (minimum) that went into preparing for the average, pre-pandemic gig (which included phone/email exchanges with the organizer about the context of the event and what they're hoping I cover, me mapping out what I want to say and how I want to present this while making sure I'm covering the organizer's requested content), plus an hour (minimum) to rehearse, plus an hour to put on makeup and get dressed, plus showing up thirty minutes early for tech check, plus an hour for the gig itself, this compensation works out to $7.69/hour, approximately half of minimum wage in Alberta. As someone who has a stable university income, I was able to comfortably (albeit with frustration) decline these offers, but it worries me that this depreciation is likely happening across the board to my fellow artists, some of whom don't have the economic security I do.

While I recognize that many organizations are facing budget cuts, the reality is that even prior to the pandemic, The Artist has seldom been fairly compensated for their labour. This is especially true for emerging artists, who don't often know how much to ask for, or who are told that poorly compensated gigs are still good opportunities to gain exposure, or who don't want to seem ungrateful or risk losing the gig by asking for a higher payment. I still rarely get invitations to gigs that mention payment in the initial offer, which implies that the person or organization reaching out doesn't value the artist's time and doesn't see being an artist as a job. Can you imagine contracting any other kind of worker and not discussing payment in the opening conversation, or at all?

To give some organizers the benefit of the doubt, artists no longer had travel or accommodations expenses for virtual gigs. But virtual gigs require artists to invest financially in equipment, including a ring light, a videocam (if your laptop doesn't have a built in one, if you own a laptop), potentially a tripod for your smartphone (if you own a smartphone), and possibly even upgrading cellular service to minimize blurring or delayed streaming. Furthermore, we no longer had in-person tech support and had to set up and manage technical issues ourselves, including during the presentation. And the physical and emotional labour required to perform effectively also hasn't decreased. If anything, I often feel that I have to work harder to connect with an audience through a camera: enunciating extra clearly to compensate for potentially poor internet connections, making more deliberate eye contact with the lens so viewers feel seen, and exuding more energy to counteract the flattening effects of online interfaces.

Not to mention that at all times while I'm presenting, I can see the blinking number that changes when attendees enter and exit the event, which, for a sensitive artist like me who is dedicated to maintaining audience attention, is immensely stressful (despite my simultaneous mental efforts to remind myself that audience members are managing all kinds of unknown responsibilities at home, including their own jobs and childcare). I heard several comments from friends who accidentally entered someone's virtual event, noticed the low audience count, cringed, and left immediately or felt pity pressured to stay. Imagine doing a live talk where there is a number flashing over your head, *that everyone in the room can see*, that broadcasts how many people are coming and going! And imagine further, that one of the main strategies to prevent audience members from leaving is to shout them out as you see them enter and to respond to their live comments (because audience members also crave to be seen the virtual space—and rightfully so), in the midst of your performance:

This next song is about...oh hey Sandy! Thanks for coming...

*This next poem is about a difficult time in my life...Greg!
I see you! Thanks for noticing my lip colour...*

In many ways, virtual gigs are a completely new job, requiring new skill sets that many artists had to teach ourselves in the midst of a crisis. It's no wonder after each event, I feel completely depleted.

So next time there's a pandemic, let's remember that a virus doesn't diminish the value of artists' labour or art itself. Artists might not be essential workers, but *art is essential*. And our work is greedily consumed. What would 2020 have been without music, TV, movies, and books?

Often the only topic of conversation we had, outside of obsessing about the pandemic, was what TV shows we were binging. Because consuming art is not only a form of escape, or a source of comfort or inspiration, it can also be a communal experience, a catalyst for connection. If we couldn't be physically together, at least we could tweet and text about *Tiger King* and the new Fiona Apple album. And sometimes, in the absence of physical hangouts, the fictional characters we regularly watched on screen became our makeshift friends, like my new *Dynasty* buds.

Personally, I found myself consuming my favourite art from the '90s—like R.E.M. albums and Winona Ryder movies—because they offered me the fun distraction of discerning if they had held up over time and how I defined holding up. They also offered me the gift of nostalgia, memories of a time full of curiosity, exploration, and most importantly, sans virus.

5
LESS SURVEILLANCE, LESS JUDGEMENT, MORE GRACE

SPEAKING OF MY FAVOURITE CHILDHOOD ART, throughout 2020, I often felt like Rachel Lynde, the town gossip from *Anne of Green Gables*, as I caught myself monitoring who was wearing masks, who was wearing them properly, and what were my neighbours doing. And I was being watched too. Being part of a queer couple (that lives together), I'm already familiar with being surveilled (and the impact of feeling unsafe even where I live), but I was still caught off guard when one of my neighbours crisply commented to me in the elevator, "You have a lot of guests over, hey?" I was too embarrassed to confess that I was living off DoorDash.

Some of this surveillance was a protective mechanism. If we watched others, we could somehow determine who to stay clear of in order to avoid potentially catching the virus. Our governments promoted this behaviour by introducing fines for transgressions and encouraging us to snitch on each other. And frankly, we were also bored. When one of my neighbours started having very loud sex in December, after being quiet for most of the year, my boyfriend and I obsessively speculated about whether he was cheating on his girlfriend or if they'd had a breakthrough in couples therapy.

Our surveillance also allowed us to feel morally superior, despite the fact that, let's face it, we all broke our share of COVID rules at some point. Our sense of moral superiority is thoroughly documented in the many think pieces that seem to come out every day, and were especially popular in the early weeks of the pandemic. While some humble bragged about the new hobbies they had taken up, the projects they had completed, and the items they had finally crossed off their long-standing task lists, others condemned the drive to be productive, while not acknowledging that, for many of us, work is a coping mechanism (sure, it's a mechanism ingrained by capitalism and perhaps one worth interrogating, but not in the midst of a global crisis). And social media shaming reached new heights as many condemned the "bad" behaviour of others (the subtext: "I would never do *that*...").

All of these forms of surveillance produced widespread and colossal guilt. Guilt seemed to be the most universal emotion in my circles. We felt guilty when we were working. We felt guilty when we weren't working. We felt guilty for complaining while others were working to provide us with the necessities of life, while others were sick. We felt guilty about breaking governmental rules that often seem arbitrary and inconsistent. We felt guilty about having privilege. When we expressed our guilt, often the best advice we had for each other was "do what you need to do to survive," and yet we didn't know how to embrace this advice without feeling guilty.

The problem with guilt is that it's a feeling that lacks movement or momentum. Unlike anger or sadness, it can't be channeled or molded. Instead, guilt hunkers down and, if anything, impedes action or change.

Next time there's a pandemic, I will try to feel less guilty. This starts by dismantling my initial question: Did I do the lockdown wrong? Maybe—for all the reasons I've shared. Or maybe not. Maybe it's not a useful question.

Because when I revisit other traumatic experiences in my life, I would never evaluate how "well" I "did" them. I got through them. I survived them. Insisting that catastrophes are teachable moments denies the severity of what happened and the aftermath. This explains why I cringed every time I heard the pandemic being referred to as an "opportunity."

Next time there's a pandemic, maybe I'll react the exact ways I did this time around. Maybe I will fare worse. Maybe I won't survive. But I hope that at least, I will offer myself, and others, more grace, more permission to flounder, to be scared, to feel hopeless, to resist comparison, to open up, and to shut down.

| In addition to these five reflections, I would like to share with you this list of commitments I scribbled in a notebook in March 2020 when I was trying to envision how we might live differently after the pandemic was "over." I invite you to repeat any of these commitments that resonate with you aloud.

We will leave our phones at home when we meet our friends.

We won't cross the street when we see someone coming towards us.

We will see conflict as an opportunity to build intimacy with those we cherish.

We will stop cancelling on each other.

We will stop cancelling each other.

We won't ask "How are you?" unless we are prepared to hear the full, honest response.

We will honour "How are you?" as an invitation for this honesty and not a reason to retreat.

We will abolish dad hugs and embrace fully.

We will honour touch as a gift.

We will create more ways and find more reasons to be in the same room with one another.

We will see and support as much live art as we can.

We will continue to spend copious amounts of time outdoors.

We will continue to wash our hands after using public washrooms.

We will continue to wear masks in public when we have a cold.

We will honour frontline workers by fighting to ensure that they earn more than minimum wage and have paid sick days.

We will never let ourselves stay too safe, too comfortable.

When we say "I hope you're well," we will mean the vast extent of wellness.

Next time there's a pandemic, what might *you* do differently? I invite you to write your own list of commitments below.

_____

_____

_____

_____

_____

_____

_____

_____

_____

_____

_____

_____

_____

_____

_____

_____

_____

_____

_____

_____

_____

_____

_____

_____

_____

_____

_____

_____

I'd like to end with a song called "Showing Up." I wrote it about my efforts to carve a new relationship with music after I realized my music dreams wouldn't come true, but it took on a new meaning in 2020. There have been so many times when I've wanted to drop out of my work, my friendships, my life, but I've been trying to find ways to keep showing up when I can and also to honour the moments when I can't.

SHOWING UP

We didn't quite make it
But we didn't quite break it
It's easy to walk away
And it's just as easy to stay

Both sides have their merits
But in any marriage
You gotta keep showing up—that's the work
You gotta keep showing up

So with every note I sing, I'm showing up
Not sure what it means but I'll keep on showing up
I might never sing outside this room
For anyone other than you
But that's enough
As long as I keep showing up

I didn't quite reach you
But you're still teaching me to
Think of our love
Beyond and outside of

Any measure
Of success or failure
You gotta keep showing up—that's the work
I gotta keep showing

So with every note I sing, I'm showing up
And it's everything that I keep on showing up
I might never strike a chord
And always feel ignored
But it's enough as long as I keep showing up.

AFTERWORD

J. R. Carpenter in Conversation with Vivek Shraya

IT SEEMS LIKE A VERY LONG TIME AGO NOW. During those early days of the first lockdown, alone in a small town in North Yorkshire, UK, endlessly scrolling through social media on my phone, news of a new book was making waves on Twitter: *The Subtweet*, by Vivek Shraya. A book about Twitter, launching on Twitter. Finally, someone writing with nuance and compassion about female friendships from inside the social media pressure cooker within which we increasingly find ourselves living out our loves, losses, desires, and ambitions. All the more so during the pandemic.

The Subtweet Virtual Book Tour events were mostly happening in far off time zones. Watching video recordings of live events after the fact, I marveled at the grace with which Vivek acknowledged and incorporated the awkwardness of the situation into her performance. Giggling nervously as an invisible audience drifts in from the far corners of the internet, "just your average awkward giggly-ness," she says, and then proceeds to introduce her leafy green houseplants by name, all whilst wearing a fabulous matching glittering green dress.

The Subtweet was the first book I ordered from Glass Bookshop when I arrived in Edmonton in August 2020. I devoured it whilst still in quarantine. When the Canadian Literature Centre asked me to introduce Vivek's Kreisel Lecture I squealed with excitement! And then panicked. How to introduce someone you've never met? And someone as multitalented as Vivek, working across music, theatre, literature, and visual art. And how not to be boring? In the early pages of *The Subtweet*, Neela offers some withering remarks on the convention of reading bios before events, featuring copious adjectives, hyperbolic comparisons, and exhaustive lists of accolades. From what I knew of her work already I had a feeling Vivek's lecture would be anything but conventional. I wondered if we could use the time traditionally afforded to reading bios a little differently. Could we have a conversation instead? A chat, even. Could we have some fun?

The following interview expands on a live conversation Vivek and I had just before her Kreisel Lecture was broadcast. I want to thank Vivek, and the CLC, for being so open to this possibility.

JRC: On the night of your Kreisel Lecture, we chatted live, just before your lecture was broadcast. I had yet to see your lecture, and you had yet to see my questions. I don't know about you, but I was nervous as heck. What made you decide you didn't want to hear the questions beforehand? What energy do you get from live interaction?

VS: Typically, a lot of rehearsal and preparation goes into any of my live events, but the Q & A portion allows me some (necessary) space for spontaneity. If I know the questions in advance, I will likely overthink my answers, and I like surprising myself, the audience, and the moderator. I feed off the interplay with the moderator, and try to create more of a conversational atmosphere because I find impromptu interaction more interesting, especially when I am an audience member.

I also welcome the chance to show the audience the cheekier, more irreverent side of me, which doesn't always come across in my performances (though ultimately, I see the Q & A as a different kind of performance). I never answer questions "for myself," as an act of self-indulgence, but always for the audience—how to keep them engaged, entertained, and challenged.

JRC: Here in print, readers may not have a sense of the how visual your lecture was. A far cry from a reading a paper at a podium, you presented us with a fully animated audio video performance experience, with outfit changes and everything. Could you set the scene for us? How did this format come about?

VS: When Interim CLC Director Sarah Krotz and I started talking about how to approach this year's lecture, the obvious choice would have been an online talk hosted on Zoom. However, when I suggested we explore a different format—one that would allow me to bring in various elements of my art practice, including music, poetry, and photography—Sarah was very encouraging. After doing numerous virtual events in 2020 and feeling generally underwhelmed (and even bored) by them, I was desperate for an opportunity to be creative. I pitched the idea of creating an animated video, and thankfully, Sarah and the CLC board said yes!

JRC: One of the questions from the audience was about the choice of the TV screen backdrop of the video lecture. Could you share your aesthetic approach and inspiration for the lecture?

VS: I have created many short films and music videos but had never recorded a lecture. Since the most popular online videos these days, like TikTok videos, are getting shorter and shorter, I knew my biggest challenge would be holding the audience's attention for twenty to thirty minutes. That said, TED Talks are also very popular and are the gold standard for online lectures, so I spent some time studying a few of them. TED Talks are shot in front of a live audience using multiple cameras, and there is usually also some kind of AV presentation in the background that the camera can cut to. Despite these advantages, they are visually a bit static (no offence to TED Talks or the speakers) and I wanted my lecture to be captivating.

I started to think beyond lectures to monologues in popular culture and recalled one of my favourite scenes in *The Matrix Reloaded* when Neo meets The Architect and he delivers a lengthy monologue while corresponding images flash on the wall of mini TV screens surrounding him. I loved the idea of working with TV screens as a backdrop because stacked TVs are simultaneously retro and futuristic, which would balance the acute time specificity of a lecture about the coronavirus pandemic. I wanted the lecture to look like it could have been created in the past, the present, or the future. Also, there was an added meta quality to featuring TV screens after a year of working, connecting, and languishing through screens.

I approached Gabriela Osio Vanden, a brilliant videographer I had collaborated on music videos with in the past, and she also loved the idea of using a TV screen backdrop. We tried to figure out how to build a wall of physical TVs, but that would have been too costly. I wasn't ready to let the idea go, and eventually we decided to use a green screen, which opened up new possibilities, including animation.

JRC: You worked with an animator to produce the video backdrop for the lecture. You've worked with illustrators and designers on your book projects as well. Why do you so often seek out collaboration?

VS: What I love about collaborating is that other artists bring their own unique perspectives to a project—perspectives that are typically quite different from my own, which ultimately results in richer, more multidimensional art. For instance, the animator of the video lecture, Tim Singleton, suggested giving each of the five reflections a distinct colour theme, pulled from SMPTE colour bars, which not only holds the audience's attention by varying the visuals, but also gives each section its own specific tone. One of my favourite animations in the video is the pairing of animated sirens with animated eyes with my comments about heightened surveillance. I would have never come up with those ideas on my own.

Collaborating with other artists also creates opportunities to learn from someone else's creative style and methods, and to build new relationships. Making art with another human is a beautiful way to create a friendship.

JRC: As I was deep-diving into your work in preparation for our conversation, I was struck by a line in your first novel, *She of the Mountains*, where you write, "White expanded limitlessly and drained every other colour out until all that could be seen was...whitewhitewhitewhitewhite."

There are so many other colours in your work, vivid bright colours which refuse to be drained away. For example, the predominant colour in Raymond Biesinger's wonderful illustrations for *She of the Mountains* is greengreengreen. Talk to me about this green. Where does it come from? Where does it take us?

VS: Much as I like being challenged when working collaboratively, I also enjoy pushing artists into new territory for them. One of the reasons I chose to work with Raymond for *She of the Mountains* is because he had never created illustrations of Hindu gods before. At the time, he also tended to work primarily in black and white, and when I scanned his website, I noticed he hadn't worked much with green in his rare colour illustrations.

Also, I can be a bit literal, and creation is a central theme in the novel. What colour says "life" more than green?

JRC: On the cover of your graphic novel, *Death Threat*, created in collaboration with Ness Lee, a blank white page cuts a brown body in half. Inside the book, the pages are anything but white. Colour works overtime, like a Greek chorus. Talk to me about how colour is saying what words can't here.

VS: Like Raymond, Ness tended to work predominantly in black and white, so I presented her with the challenge of using colour. This was also important to me because I worried a book called *Death Threat* and illustrated in black and white would feel dire and smother the humour at the core of project. Colour, however, can be overwhelming, especially in the often maximalist world of graphic novels. We agreed it would be more manageable to come up with a specific colour palette for the book. My biggest aesthetic inspiration for this project was artist Ricardo Avolo's work, which often features primary colours. I also loved how our use of primary colours reclaims them from iconic, masculine-centric comics like *Superman*, and uses them to tell a trans feminine narrative.

JRC: In *Death Threat,* and in many of your other works, you take on huge topics with relatively few words. Talk to me about how you work with sparsity in you prose. Does working with illustrators enable you to say more with less?

VS: For me, including illustrations is another means of inviting a reader into the text. Also, I'm not a verbose writer. I strive to be as concise as possible. Working with illustrators is an opportunity to have the text be revealed beyond words and even redirected beyond the meaning I intended.

JRC: There's a line in *I'm Afraid of Men* where you write, "Before every gig, Nick helped me choose which dress, what lipstick colour (I taught him my favourite shade names)."

I've seen you in a fair few Zoom gigs now. I'm always impressed with just how considered those choices are. Not only did the green dress of *The Subtweet* Virtual Book Tour shimmer amid the lustrous leaves of your giant house plants, but those same green leaves are echoed on the cover of the book itself! Before our live chat before the Kreisel Lecture, I asked you what we should wear on Zoom. You said, something fashionably futuristic. I thought, wow! This is conceptual art.

Can you elaborate a bit more on the critical thinking that goes into these choices? How are you extending conceptual and aesthetic themes in your work into the world, communicating through colour, wardrobe, make-up?

VS: As a queer, POC artist who lacked institutional support for over half of my career, I've had to be hyper creative to draw audiences to my art. Beginning my art practice as a pop musician, I learned how pivotal aesthetic is in establishing connection—a song is never enough on its own. I invest a lot time in considering the potential visual aspects of every project—from the font and artwork, to press photos, to video teasers, to tour uniform. I don't see these aspects as separate from the art because in addition to attracting audiences, they can also enhance their engagement with the art itself. A press photo can be more than a press photo: it can also amplify the story inherent in the project that it's being used to promote.

This is why I strongly oppose the ways aesthetic is dismissed as superficial because this—often sexist—trivialization actually speaks to a missed opportunity to extend the art itself, and diminishes the work involved in creative direction.

JRC: I totally agree. In your collection of short stories, *God Loves Hair*, we get a sense of just how deep those aesthetic preoccupations run. In a story called "Lipstick" you write, "All the bright colours are dazzling. But I am greedy for the colours that hide, the glossy surprises caged within lipstick shells. They call to me. One by one, I remove their lids, twist the blushing sticks to the top, smear my face like oil on canvas. Then I smash the lids back on, completely crushing the lipsticks." Do you think a creative writing course on coming up with good make-up names would be better taught at undergraduate or graduate level?

VS: This would definitely be a fun writing prompt in an undergraduate creative writing class, but I would also welcome the opportunity to work with a graduate student who wanted to write a paper on the history of make-up names.

JRC: Could we could just take a moment to appreciate the cover design of *I'm Afraid of Men*? I think this is the book of yours I would most like to wear. Talk to me about these colour choices.

VS: Having a long-term colourful aesthetic poses the challenge of how to differentiate each new design from my other projects. The book designer, Jennifer Griffiths, selected these colours, perhaps in part because they aren't a colour palette I've used in previous projects. My other ask was that we avoid any on-the-nose "gender colours" for this book, like blue and pink.

JRC: Talk to me about the back cover, and its relationship with the front cover. Talk to me about the period. At the end of the title.

VS: The book cover and design are so important and not just because I learnt from self-publishing my first book, *God Loves Hair*, that people *do* judge a book by its cover, but also because I see the book itself as a public art object, especially when you consider the how often books are read in public. So I loved when my editor, David Ross, suggested that we print the line "Men Are Afraid of Me" from my conclusion on the back cover. First, it enhances the meaning of the title. On its own, "I'm afraid of men" can read as a vulnerable and even irrational, but the visual juxtaposition with "men are afraid me" on the back cover asserts that my fear isn't just neurotic or random but stems from an unacknowledged reality: men's discomfort with me. Second, when read in public, the front and back cover can act as a talisman and a tangible form of resistance for women and feminine people. Also, while it's easy for men to become defensive when they initially see (or hear) the title, when the back cover invites them to reflect and be accountable, if they choose.

The period was the designer's choice, and I think that it makes the title less of a comment someone might say in passing, like "I'm afraid of heights," and more of a declaration that you might see on a protest poster.

JRC: In your poetry collection, *even this page is white*, you write, "even / this page / is white / so I protest this page." If you could write a book on any colour paper, what colour would you choose?

VS: A colour that is warm and inviting, like yellow. Aside: I'm still dreaming of a gold book cover!

JRC: One of the many things I love about *even this page is white* is white is the decision to ground the text at the bottom of the pages so that the white space is something the reader has to, well, read, before getting to the text.

VS: The title *even this page is white* required me to consider the page not just figuratively but also literally. I wanted to show on the page how people of colour are always pushed to the margins (there I go being literal again!) and yet, despite this, we are still here. We can't be completely erased. I also reclaim the page fully at the end of the book (spoiler) by situating the final poem, "brown dreams," squarely in the centre.

JRC: Following hot on the heels of *The Subtweet* Virtual Book Tour you recently launched a third book during lockdown, *How to Fail as a Popstar*, based on your play of the same name. For the online launch event, you colour-coordinated your eyeshadow to match the book cover. This got me wondering: Which would you rather host: a reality TV show on makeovers, or a reality TV show on interior decoration?

VS: All of the above please! Confession: I LOVE home renovation shows. One of my pandemic binges was Netflix's *Marriage or Mortgage*. Clearly, I should host the second season.

JRC: Clearly! In your lecture you talk about the unreasonable expectation of productivity many of us struggled with during the pandemic, so I'm not going to ask what you worked on during lockdown, but curious to know how slowly coming out of lockdown has altered the way you work or think about your work.

VS: The pandemic has really reaffirmed for me my love for collaboration. In many ways, I've been forced to be a "solo artist" this past year, and while I can do it, and sometimes, like with writing, it's a necessity, it's not how I thrive. Solo = boring. So, before the next pandemic, I hope to create a fuck ton of art with other artists!

And in the meantime, I'm so grateful for this thoughtful dialogue with you, J. R.

ACKNOWLEDGEMENTS

THANK YOU, Shemeena Shraya, Adam Holman, Trisha Yeo, J. R. Carpenter, Sarah Krotz, Jason Purcell, Marie Carrière, Gabriela Osio Vanden, Tim Singleton, Michelle Lobkowicz, Joanne Muzak, and the University of Alberta Press team.

The CBC article referenced is by Stephanie Hogan: "This Is Your Brain on Pandemic: What Chronic Stress Is Doing to Us," *CBC News*, April 1, 2021, https://www.cbc.ca/news/health/pandemic-brain-stress-effect-lethargy-unproductive-1.5972055.

CLC KREISEL LECTURE SERIES

Published by University of Alberta Press and the Canadian Literature Centre / Centre de littérature canadienne